Slow Cooker Breakfast Cookbook for Women Over 50

Easy, Delicious, Healthy Recipes For Every Breakfast of the Day!

By Karen Epstein

© **Copyright 2021 - All rights reserved.**

The content contained within this book may not be reproduced, duplicated or transmitted without direct written permission from the author or the publisher.

Under no circumstances will any blame or legal responsibility be held against the publisher, or author, for any damages, reparation, or monetary loss due to the information contained within this book. Either directly or indirectly.

Legal Notice:

This book is copyright protected. This book is only for personal use. You cannot amend, distribute, sell, use, quote or paraphrase any part, or the content within this book, without the consent of the author or publisher.

Disclaimer Notice:

Please note the information contained within this document is for educational and entertainment purposes only. All effort has been executed to present accurate, up to date, and reliable, complete information. No warranties of any kind are declared or implied. Readers acknowledge that the author is not engaging in the rendering of legal, financial, medical or professional advice. The content within this book has been derived from various sources. Please consult a licensed professional before attempting any techniques outlined in this book.

By reading this document, the reader agrees that under no circumstances is the author responsible for any losses, direct or indirect, which are incurred as a result of the use of information contained within this document, including, but not limited to, — errors, omissions, or inaccuracies.

Sommario

Slow Cooker Breakfast Recipes 9
Oats Granola 9
Chili Eggs Mix 11
Tropical Granola 14
Cheesy Eggs 16
Creamy Strawberries Oatmeal 18
Tomato and Zucchini Eggs Mix 20
Breakfast Potatoes 22
Chocolate Breakfast Bread 24
Hash Brown Mix 27
Almond and Quinoa Bowls 29
Bacon and Egg Casserole 31
Carrots Casserole 33
Breakfast Rice Pudding 35
Cranberry Maple Oatmeal 37
Apple Breakfast Rice 40
Mushroom Casserole 42
Quinoa and Banana Mix 44
Ginger Apple Bowls 46
Dates Quinoa 48
Granola Bowls 50
Cinnamon Quinoa 53
Squash Bowls 55
Quinoa and Apricots 57
Lamb and Eggs Mix 59

Blueberry Quinoa Oatmeal	61
Cauliflower Casserole	63
Lentils and Quinoa Mix	66
Beef Meatloaf	68
Butternut Squash Quinoa	70
Leek Casserole	72
Chia Seeds Mix	74
Eggs and Sweet Potato Mix	76
Chia Seeds and Chicken Breakfast	79
Pork and Eggplant Casserole	81
Chocolate Quinoa	83
Apple Spread	85
Chai Breakfast Quinoa	87
Cherries and Cocoa Oats	89
Quinoa Breakfast Bake	92
Beans Salad	94
Mocha Latte Quinoa Mix	96
Peppers Rice Mix	98
Breakfast Butterscotch Pudding	100
Cashew Butter	102
French Breakfast Pudding	105
Pumpkin and Berries Bowls	107
Eggs and Sausage Casserole	109
Quinoa and Chia Pudding	111
Cauliflower Rice Pudding	113
Beans Breakfast Bowls	115

Conclusion... 119

Introduction

We know you are always searching for simpler ways to prepare your meals. We also understand you are most likely tired investing long hours in the kitchen cooking with many frying pans and also pots.

Well, now your search mores than! We located the ideal kitchen device you can make use of from now on! We are speaking about the Slow cooker! These outstanding pots enable you to prepare a few of the best recipes ever with minimal effort Slow-moving stoves prepare your meals less complicated and a lot much healthier! You do not require to be a specialist in the kitchen to cook some of one of the most scrumptious, flavored, textured as well as abundant recipes!
All you require is your Slow cooker and the ideal active ingredients! This great recipe book you will find will teach you exactly how to prepare the very best slow prepared meals. It will reveal you that you can make some outstanding breakfasts, lunch meals, side recipes, fowl, meat as well as fish meals. Ultimately yet importantly, this recipe book offers you some basic as well as wonderful desserts.

Slow Cooker Breakfast Recipes

Oats Granola

Preparation time: 10 minutes

Cooking time: 2 hours

Servings: 8

Ingredients:

- 5 cups old-fashioned rolled oats
- 1/3 cup coconut oil
- 2/3 cup honey
- ½ cup almonds, chopped
- ½ cup peanut butter
- 1 tablespoon vanilla

- 2 teaspoons cinnamon powder

- 1 cup craisins

- Cooking spray

Directions:

1. Grease your Slow cooker with cooking spray, add oats, oil, honey, almonds, peanut butter, vanilla, craisins and cinnamon, toss just a bit, cover and cook on High for 2 hours, stirring every 30 minutes.

2. Divide into bowls and serve for breakfast.

Nutrition: calories 200, fat 3, fiber 6, carbs 9, protein 4

Chili Eggs Mix

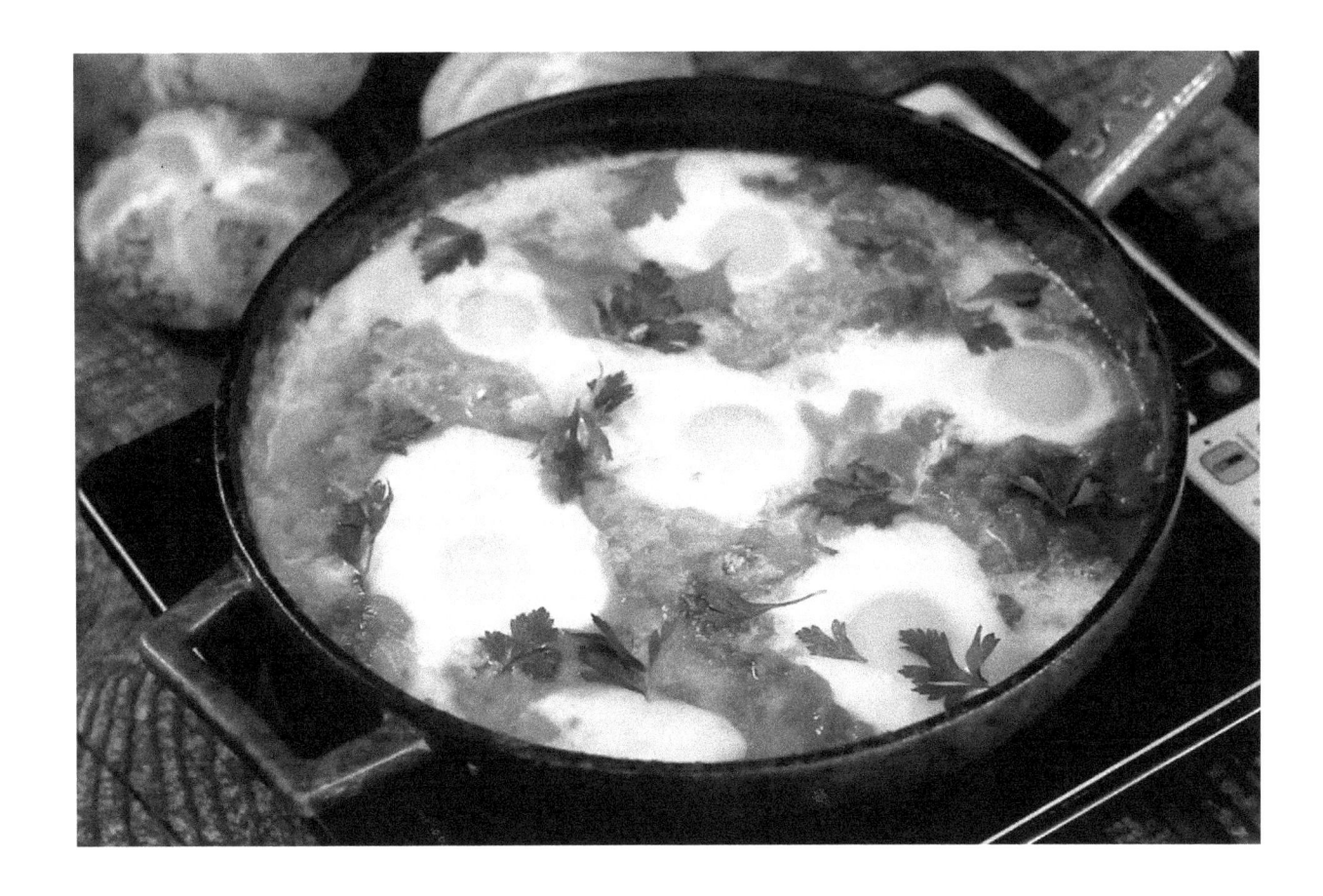

Preparation time: 10 minutes

Cooking time: 3 hours

Servings: 2

Ingredients:

- Cooking spray
- 3 spring onions, chopped
- 2 tablespoons sun dried tomatoes, chopped
- 1 ounce canned and roasted green chili pepper, chopped
- ½ teaspoon rosemary, dried
- Salt and black pepper to the taste
- 3 ounces cheddar cheese, shredded
- 4 eggs, whisked
- ¼ cup heavy cream
- 1 tablespoon chives, chopped

Directions:

1. Grease your slow cooker with cooking spray and mix the eggs with the chili peppers and the other ingredients except the cheese.

2. Toss everything into the pot, sprinkle the cheese on top, put the lid on and cook on High for 3 hours.

3. Divide between plates and serve.

Nutrition: calories 224, fat 4, fiber 7, carbs 18, protein 11

Tropical Granola

Preparation time: 10 minutes

Cooking time: 1 hour and 30 minutes

Servings: 6

Ingredients:

- 1 cup almonds, sliced
- 4 cups old-fashioned oats
- ½ cup pecans, chopped
- ½ teaspoon ginger, ground
- ½ cup coconut oil
- ½ cup dried coconut
- ½ cup raisins
- ½ cup dried cherries

- ½ cup pineapple, dried

Directions:

1. In your Slow cooker, mix oil with almonds, oats, pecans, ginger, coconut, raisins, cherries and pineapple, toss, cover, cook on High for 1 hour and 30 minutes, stir again, divide into bowls and serve for breakfast.

Nutrition: calories 172, fat 5, fiber 8, carbs 10, protein 4

Cheesy Eggs

Preparation time: 10 minutes

Cooking time: 3 hours

Servings: 2

Ingredients:

- 4 eggs, whisked
- ¼ cup spring onions, chopped
- 1 tablespoon oregano, chopped
- 1 cup milk
- 2 ounces feta cheese, crumbled
- A pinch of salt and black pepper
- Cooking spray

Directions:

1. In a bowl, combine the eggs with the spring onions and the other ingredients except the cooking spray and whisk.

2. Grease your slow cooker with cooking spray, add eggs mix, stir , put the lid on and cook on Low for 3 hours.

3. Divide between plates and serve for breakfast.

Nutrition: calories 214, fat 4, fiber 7, carbs 18, protein 5

Creamy Strawberries Oatmeal

Preparation time: 10 minutes

Cooking time: 8 hours

Servings: 8

Ingredients:

- 6 cups water
- 2 cups milk
- 2 cups steel cut oats
- 1 cup Greek yogurt
- 1 teaspoon cinnamon powder
- 2 cups strawberries, halved
- 1 teaspoon vanilla extract

Directions:

1. In your Slow cooker, mix water with milk, oats, yogurt, cinnamon, strawberries and vanilla, toss, cover and cook on Low for 8 hours.

2. Divide into bowls and serve for breakfast.

Nutrition: calories 200, fat 4, fiber 6, carbs 8, protein 4

Tomato and Zucchini Eggs Mix

Preparation time: 10 minutes

Cooking time: 3 hours

Servings: 2

Ingredients:

- Cooking spray
- 4 eggs, whisked
- 2 spring onions, chopped
- 1 tablespoon basil, chopped
- ½ teaspoon turmeric powder
- ½ cup tomatoes, cubed
- 1 zucchini, grated
- ¼ teaspoon sweet paprika

- A pinch of salt and black pepper

- 1 tablespoon parsley, chopped

- 2 tablespoons parmesan, grated

Directions:

1. Grease your slow cooker with cooking spray, add the eggs mixed with the zucchini, tomatoes and the other ingredients except the cheese and stir well.

2. Sprinkle the cheese, put the lid on and cook on High for 3 hours.

3. Divide between plates and serve for breakfast right away.

Nutrition: calories 261, fat 5, fiber 7, carbs 19, protein 6

Breakfast Potatoes

Preparation time: 10 minutes

Cooking time: 4 hours

Servings: 8

Ingredients:

- 3 potatoes, peeled and cubed
- 1 green bell pepper, chopped
- 1 red bell pepper, chopped
- 1 yellow onion, chopped
- 12 ounces smoked chicken sausage, sliced
- 1 and ½ cups cheddar cheese, shredded
- ¼ teaspoon oregano, dried
- ½ cup sour cream

- ¼ teaspoon basil, dried

- 10 ounces cream of chicken soup

- 2 tablespoons parsley, chopped

- Salt and black pepper to the taste

Directions:

1. In your Slow cooker, mix potatoes with red bell pepper, green bell pepper, sausage, onion, oregano, basil, cheese, salt, pepper and cream of chicken, cover and cook on Low for 4 hours.

2. Add parsley, divide between plates and serve for breakfast.

Nutrition: calories 320, fat 5, fiber 7, carbs 10, protein 5

Chocolate Breakfast Bread

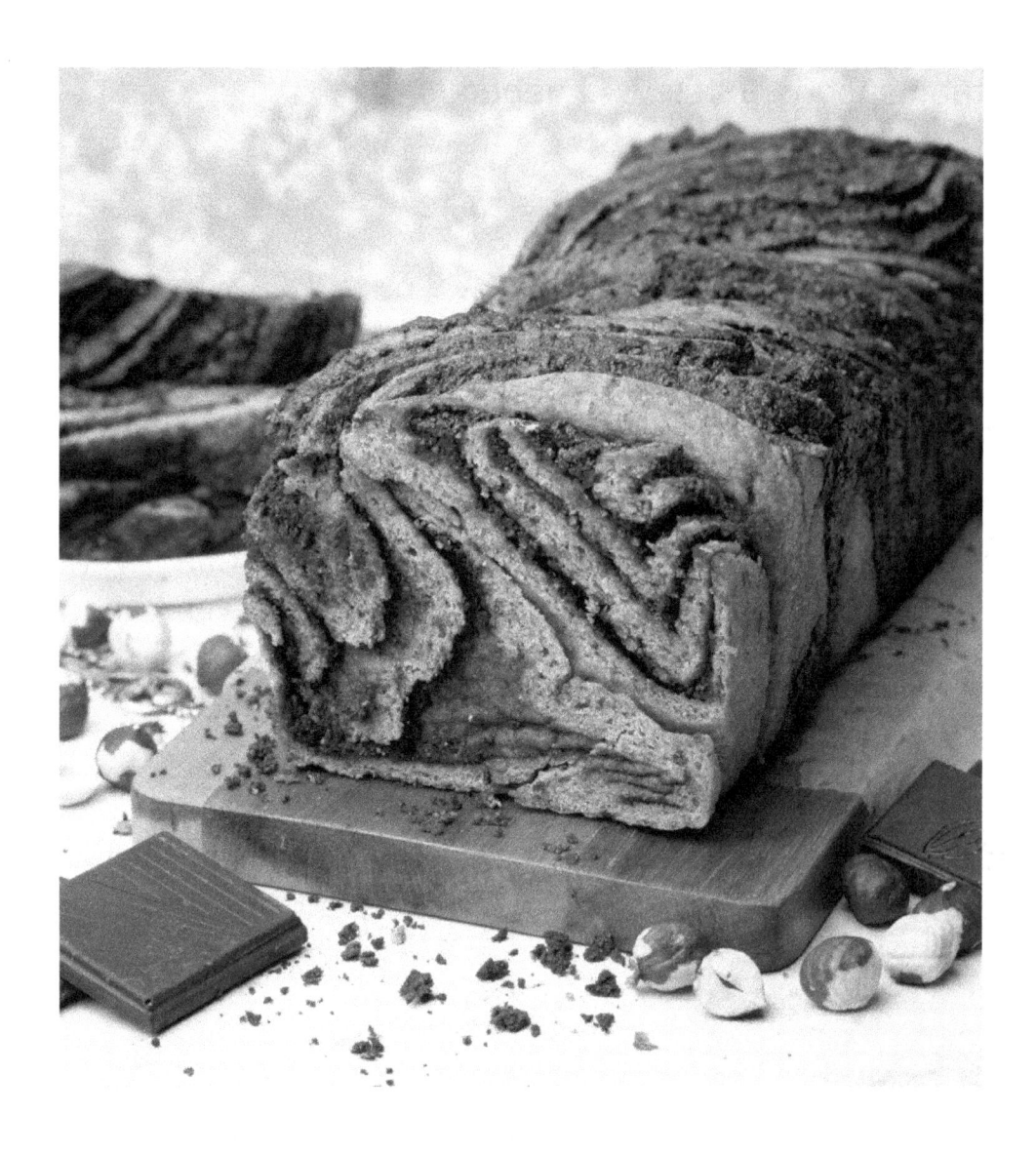

Preparation time: 10 minutes

Cooking time: 3 hours

Servings: 2

Ingredients:

- Cooking spray
- 1 cup almond flour
- ½ teaspoon baking soda
- ½ teaspoon cinnamon powder
- 1 tablespoon avocado oil
- 2 tablespoons maple syrup
- 2 eggs, whisked
- 1 tablespoon butter
- ½ tablespoon milk
- ½ teaspoon vanilla extract
- ½ cup dark chocolate, melted
- 2 tablespoons walnuts, chopped

Directions:

1. In a bowl, mix the flour with the baking soda, cinnamon, oil and the other ingredients except the cooking spray and stir well.

2. Grease a loaf pan that fits the slow cooker with the cooking spray, pour the bread batter into the pan, put the pan in the slow cooker after you've lined it with tin foil, put the lid on and cook on High for 3 hours.

3. Cool the sweet bread down, slice, divide between plates and serve for breakfast.

Nutrition: calories 200, fat 3, fiber 5, carbs 8, protein 4

Hash Brown Mix

Preparation time: 10 minutes

Cooking time: 3 hours

Servings: 6

Ingredients:

- 3 tablespoons butter
- ½ cup sour cream
- ¼ cup mushrooms, sliced
- ¼ teaspoon garlic powder
- ¼ cup yellow onion, chopped
- 1 cup milk
- 3 tablespoons flour
- 20 ounces hash browns

- Salt and black pepper to the taste

- 1 cup cheddar cheese, shredded

- Cooking spray

Directions:

1. Heat up a pan with the butter over medium-high heat, add mushrooms, onion and garlic powder, stir and cook for a few minutes.

2. Add flour and whisk well.

3. Add milk, stir really well and transfer everything to your Slow cooker greased with cooking spray.

4. Add hash browns, salt, pepper, sour cream and cheese, toss, cover and cook on High for 3 hours.

5. Divide between plates and serve for breakfast.

Nutrition: calories 262, fat 6, fiber 4, carbs 12, protein 6

Almond and Quinoa Bowls

Preparation time: 10 minutes

Cooking time: 5 hours

Servings: 2

Ingredients:

- 1 cup quinoa
- 2 cups almond milk
- 2 tablespoons butter, melted
- 2 tablespoons brown sugar
- A pinch of cinnamon powder
- A pinch of nutmeg, ground
- ¼ cup almonds, sliced
- Cooking spray

Directions:

1. Grease your slow cooker with the cooking spray, add the quinoa, milk, melted butter and the other ingredients, toss, put the lid on and cook on Low for 5 hours.

2. Divide the mix into bowls and serve for breakfast.

Nutrition: calories 211, fat 3, fiber 6, carbs 12, protein 5

Bacon and Egg Casserole

Preparation time: 10 minutes

Cooking time: 5 hours

Servings: 8

Ingredients:

- 20 ounces hash browns
- Cooking spray
- 8 ounces cheddar cheese, shredded
- 8 bacon slices, cooked and chopped
- 6 green onions, chopped
- ½ cup milk
- 12 eggs
- Salt and black pepper to the taste

- Salsa for serving

Directions:

1. Grease your Slow cooker with cooking spray, spread hash browns, cheese, bacon and green onions and toss.

2. In a bowl, mix the eggs with salt, pepper and milk and whisk really well.

3. Pour this over hash browns, cover and cook on Low for 5 hours.

4. Divide between plates and serve with salsa on top.

Nutrition: calories 300, fat 5, fiber 5, carbs 9, protein 5

Carrots Casserole

Preparation time: 10 minutes

Cooking time: 3 hours

Servings: 2

Ingredients:

- 1 teaspoon ginger, ground
- ½ pound carrots, peeled and grated
- 2 eggs, whisked
- ½ teaspoon garlic powder
- ½ teaspoon rosemary, dried
- Salt and black pepper to the taste
- 1 red onion, chopped
- 1 tablespoons parsley, chopped

- 2 garlic cloves, minced
- ½ tablespoon olive oil

Directions:

1. Grease your slow cooker with the oil and mix the carrots with the eggs, ginger and the other ingredients inside.
2. Toss, put the lid on, cook High for 3 hours, divide between plates and serve.

Nutrition: calories 218, fat 6, fiber 6, carbs 14, protein 5

Breakfast Rice Pudding

Preparation time: 10 minutes

Cooking time: 4 hours

Servings: 4

Ingredients:

- 1 cup coconut milk
- 2 cups water
- 1 cup almond milk
- ½ cup raisins
- 1 cup brown rice
- 2 teaspoons vanilla extract
- 2 tablespoons flaxseed
- 1 teaspoon cinnamon powder

- 2 tablespoons coconut sugar
- Cooking spray

Directions:

1. Grease your Slow cooker with the cooking spray, add coconut milk, water, almond milk, raisins, rice, vanilla, flaxseed and cinnamon, cover, cook on Low for 4 hours, stir, divide into bowls, sprinkle coconut sugar all over and serve.

Nutrition: calories 213, fat 3, fiber 6, carbs 10, protein 4

Cranberry Maple Oatmeal

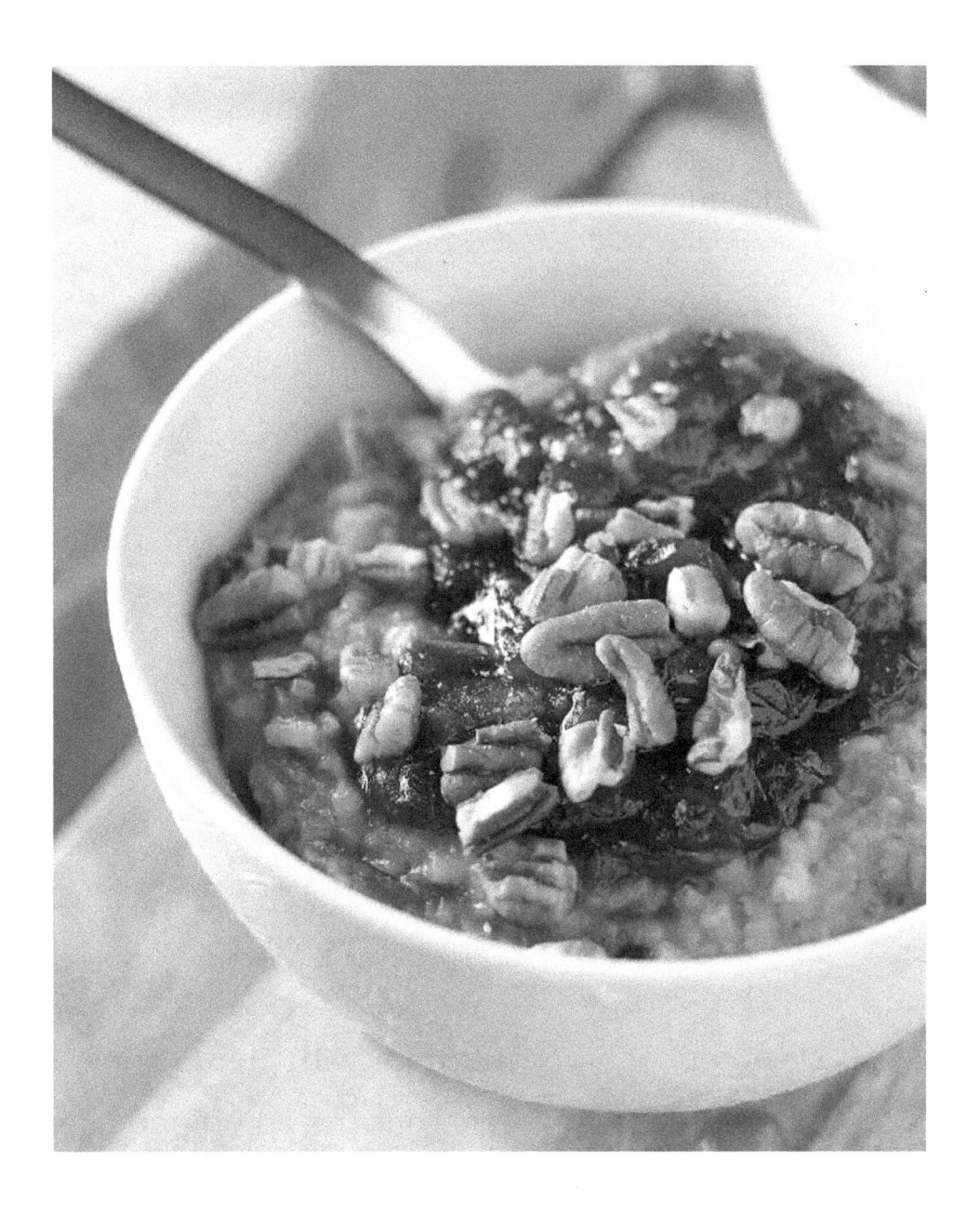

Preparation time: 10 minutes

Cooking time: 6 hours

Servings: 2

Ingredients:

- 1 cup almond milk
- ½ cup steel cut oats
- ½ cup cranberries
- ½ teaspoon vanilla extract
- 1 tablespoon maple syrup
- 1 tablespoon sugar

Directions:

1. In your slow cooker, mix the oats with the berries, milk and the other ingredients, toss, put the lid on and cook on Low for 6 hours.

2. Divide into bowls and serve for breakfast.

Nutrition: calories 200, fat 5, fiber 7, carbs 14, protein 4

Apple Breakfast Rice

Preparation time: 10 minutes

Cooking time: 7 hours

Servings: 4

Ingredients:

- 4 apples, cored, peeled and chopped
- 2 tablespoons butter
- 2 teaspoons cinnamon powder
- 1 and ½ cups brown rice
- ½ teaspoon vanilla extract
- A pinch of nutmeg, ground
- 5 cups milk

Directions:

1. Put the butter in your Slow cooker, add apples, cinnamon, rice, vanilla, nutmeg and milk, cover, cook on Low for 7 hours, stir, divide into bowls and serve for breakfast.

Nutrition: calories 214, fat 4, fiber 5, carbs 7, protein 4

Mushroom Casserole

Preparation time: 10 minutes

Cooking time: 5 hours

Servings: 2

Ingredients:

- ½ cup mozzarella, shredded
- 2 eggs, whisked
- ½ tablespoon balsamic vinegar
- ½ tablespoon olive oil
- 4 ounces baby kale
- 1 red onion, chopped
- ¼ teaspoon oregano
- ½ pound white mushrooms, sliced

- Salt and black pepper to the taste

- Cooking spray

Directions:

1. In a bowl, mix the eggs with the kale, mushrooms and the other ingredients except the cheese and cooking spray and stir well.

2. Grease your slow cooker with cooking spray, add the mushroom mix, spread, sprinkle the mozzarella all over, put the lid on and cook on Low for 5 hours.

3. Divide between plates and serve for breakfast.

Nutrition: calories 216, fat 6, fiber 8, carbs 12, protein 4

Quinoa and Banana Mix

Preparation time: 10 minutes

Cooking time: 6 hours

Servings: 8

Ingredients:

- 2 cups quinoa
- 2 bananas, mashed
- 4 cups water
- 2 cups blueberries
- 2 teaspoons vanilla extract
- 2 tablespoons maple syrup
- 1 teaspoon cinnamon powder
- Cooking spray

Directions:

1. Grease your Slow cooker with cooking spray, add quinoa, bananas, water, blueberries, vanilla, maple syrup and cinnamon, stir, cover and cook on Low for 6 hours.

2. Stir again, divide into bowls and serve for breakfast.

Nutrition: calories 200, fat 4, fiber 6, carbs 12, protein 4

Ginger Apple Bowls

Preparation time: 10 minutes

Cooking time: 6 hours

Servings: 2

Ingredients:

- 2 apples, cored, peeled and cut into medium chunks
- 1 tablespoon sugar
- 1 tablespoon ginger, grated
- 1 cup heavy cream
- ¼ teaspoon cinnamon powder
- ½ teaspoon vanilla extract
- ¼ teaspoon cardamom, ground

Directions:

1. In your slow cooker, combine the apples with the sugar, ginger and the other ingredients, toss, put the lid on and cook on Low for 6 hours.

2. Divide into bowls and serve for breakfast.

Nutrition: calories 201, fat 3, fiber 7, carbs 19, protein 4

Dates Quinoa

Preparation time: 10 minutes

Cooking time: 3 hours

Servings: 4

Ingredients:

- 1 cup quinoa
- 4 medjol dates, chopped
- 3 cups milk
- 1 apple, cored and chopped
- ¼ cup pepitas
- 2 teaspoons cinnamon powder
- 1 teaspoon vanilla extract
- ¼ teaspoon nutmeg, ground

Directions:

1. In your Slow cooker, mix quinoa with dates, milk, apple, pepitas, cinnamon, nutmeg and vanilla, stir, cover and cook on High for 3 hours.

2. Stir again, divide into bowls and serve.

Nutrition: calories 241, fat 4, fiber 4, carbs 10, protein 3

Granola Bowls

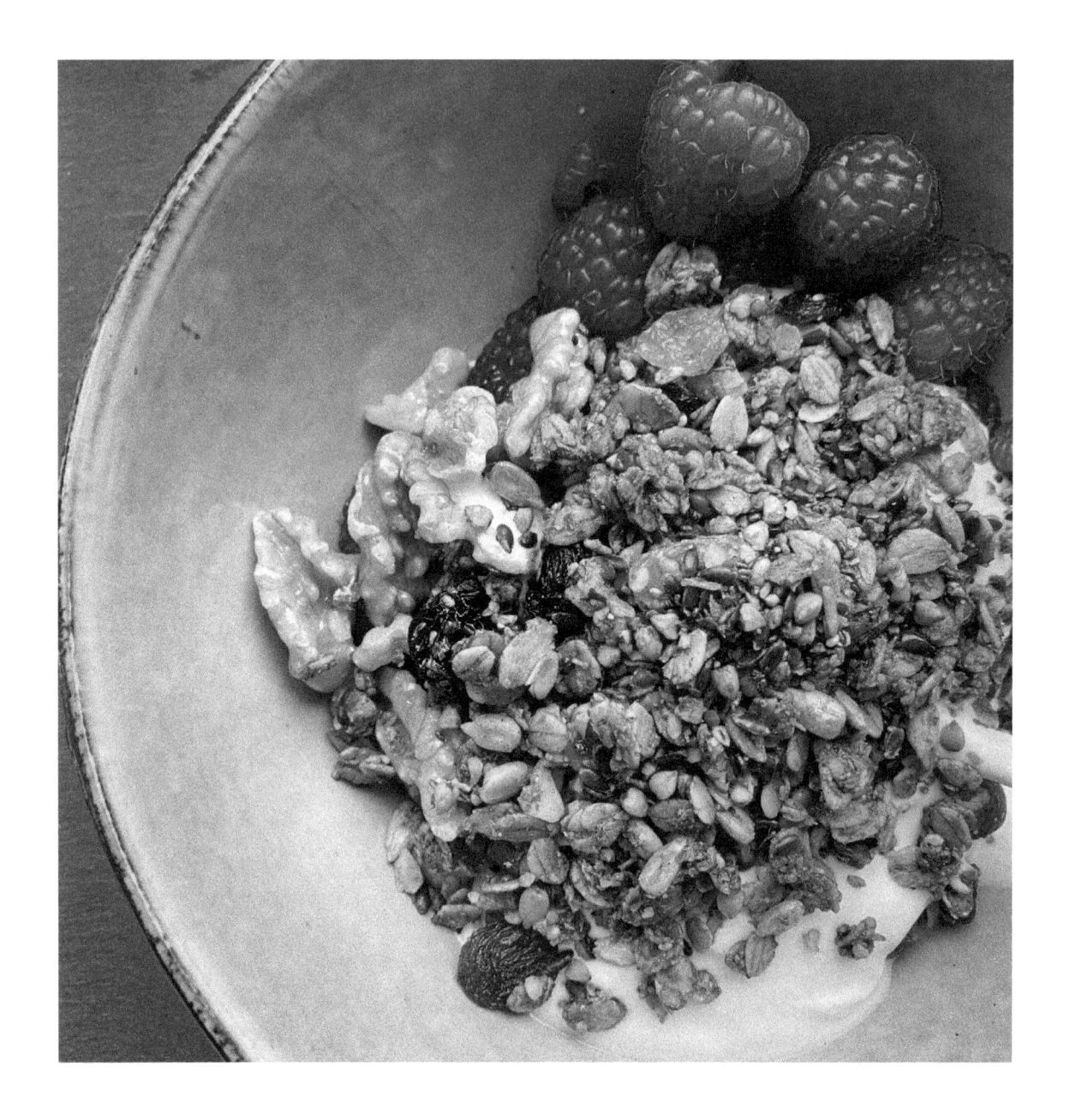

Preparation time: 10 minutes

Cooking time: 4 hours

Servings: 2

Ingredients:

- ½ cup granola
- ¼ cup coconut cream
- 2 tablespoons brown sugar
- 2 tablespoons cashew butter
- 1 teaspoon cinnamon powder
- ½ teaspoon nutmeg, ground

Directions:

1. In your slow cooker, mix the granola with the cream, sugar and the other ingredients, toss, put the lid on and cook on Low for 4 hours.

2. Divide into bowls and serve for breakfast.

Nutrition: calories 218, fat 6, fiber 9, carbs 17, protein 6

Cinnamon Quinoa

Preparation time: 10 minutes

Cooking time: 4 hours

Servings: 4

Ingredients:

- 1 cup quinoa
- 2 cups milk
- 2 cups water
- ¼ cup stevia
- 1 teaspoon cinnamon powder
- 1 teaspoon vanilla extract

Directions:

1. In your Slow cooker, mix quinoa with milk, water, stevia, cinnamon and vanilla, stir, cover, cook on Low for 3 hours and 30 minutes, stir, cook for 30 minutes more, divide into bowls and serve for breakfast.

Nutrition: calories 172, fat 4, fiber 3, carbs 8, protein 2

Squash Bowls

Preparation time: 10 minutes

Cooking time: 6 hours

Servings: 2

Ingredients:

- 2 tablespoons walnuts, chopped
- 2 cups squash, peeled and cubed
- ½ cup coconut cream
- ½ teaspoon cinnamon powder
- ½ tablespoon sugar

Directions:

1. In your slow cooker, mix the squash with the nuts and the other ingredients, toss, put the lid on and cook on Low for 6 hours.

2. Divide into bowls and serve.

Nutrition: calories 140, fat 1, fiber 2, carbs 2, protein 5

Quinoa and Apricots

Preparation time: 10 minutes

Cooking time: 10 hours

Servings: 6

Ingredients:

- ¾ cup quinoa
- ¾ cup steel cut oats
- 2 tablespoons honey
- 1 cup apricots, chopped
- 6 cups water
- 1 teaspoon vanilla extract
- ¾ cup hazelnuts, chopped

Directions:

1. In your Slow cooker, mix quinoa with oats honey, apricots, water, vanilla and hazelnuts, stir, cover and cook on Low for 10 hours.

2. Stir quinoa mix again, divide into bowls and serve for breakfast.

Nutrition: calories 200, fat 3, fiber 5, carbs 8, protein 6

Lamb and Eggs Mix

Preparation time: 10 minutes

Cooking time: 6 hours

Servings: 2

Ingredients:

- 1 pound lamb meat, ground
- 4 eggs, whisked
- 1 tablespoon basil, chopped
- ½ teaspoon cumin powder
- 1 tablespoon chili powder
- 1 red onion, chopped
- 1 tablespoon olive oil
- A pinch of salt and black pepper

Directions:

1. Grease the slow cooker with the oil and mix the lamb with the eggs, basil and the other ingredients inside.

2. Toss, put the lid on, cook on Low for 6 hours, divide into bowls and serve for breakfast.

Nutrition: calories 220, fat 2, fiber 2, carbs 6, protein 2

Blueberry Quinoa Oatmeal

Preparation time: 10 minutes

Cooking time: 8 hours

Servings: 4

Ingredients:

- ½ cup quinoa
- 1 cup steel cut oats
- 1 teaspoon vanilla extract
- 5 cups water
- Zest of 1 lemon, grated
- 1 teaspoon vanilla extract
- 2 tablespoons flaxseed
- 1 tablespoon butter, melted

- 3 tablespoons maple syrup

- 1 cup blueberries

Directions:

1. In your Slow cooker, mix butter with quinoa, water, oats, vanilla, lemon zest, flaxseed, maple syrup and blueberries, stir, cover and cook on Low for 8 hours.

2. Divide into bowls and serve for breakfast.

Nutrition: calories 189, fat 5, fiber 5, carbs 20, protein 5

Cauliflower Casserole

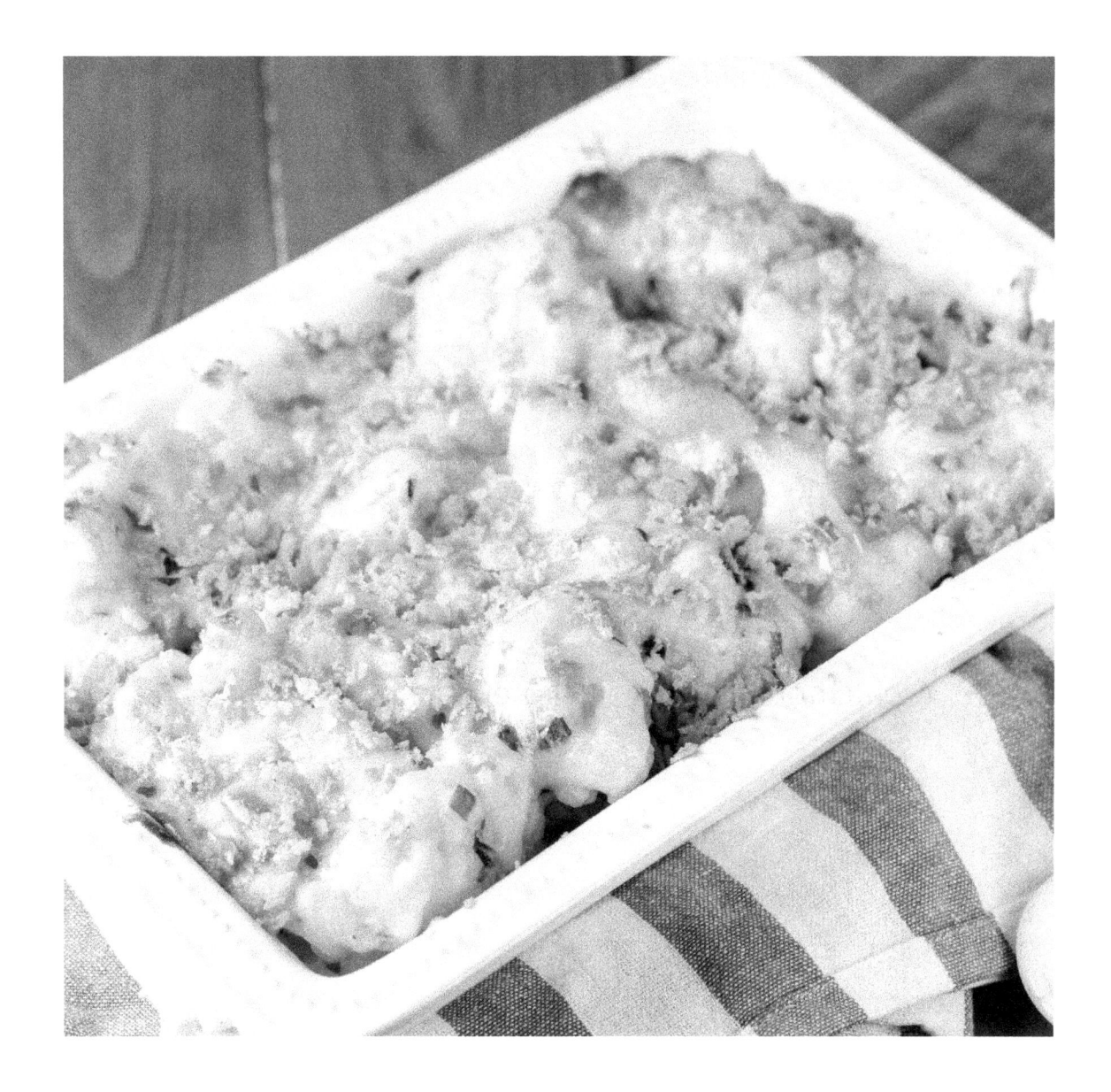

Preparation time: 10 minutes

Cooking time: 5 hours

Servings: 2

Ingredients:

- 1 pound cauliflower florets
- 3 eggs, whisked
- 1 red onion, sliced
- ½ teaspoon sweet paprika
- ½ teaspoon turmeric powder
- 1 garlic clove, minced
- A pinch of salt and black pepper
- Cooking spray

Directions:

1. Spray your slow cooker with the cooking spray, and mix the cauliflower with the eggs, onion and the other ingredients inside.

2. Put the lid on, cook on Low for 5 hours, divide between 2 plates and serve for breakfast.

Nutrition: calories 200, fat 3, fiber 6, carbs 13, protein 8

Lentils and Quinoa Mix

Preparation time: 10 minutes

Cooking time: 8 hours

Servings: 6

Ingredients:

- 3 garlic cloves, minced
- 1 yellow onion, chopped
- 1 celery stalk, chopped
- 2 red bell peppers, chopped
- 12 ounces canned tomatoes, chopped
- 4 cups veggie stock
- 1 cup lentils
- 14 ounces pinto beans

- 2 tablespoons chili powder

- ½ cup quinoa

- 1 tablespoons oregano, chopped

- 2 teaspoon cumin, ground

Directions:

1. In your Slow cooker, mix garlic with the onion, celery, bell peppers, tomatoes, stock, lentils, pinto beans, chili powder, quinoa, oregano and cumin, stir, cover, cook on Low for 8 hours, divide between plates and serve for breakfast

Nutrition: calories 231, fat 4, fiber 5, carbs 16, protein 4

Beef Meatloaf

Preparation time: 10 minutes

Cooking time: 4 hours

Servings: 2

Ingredients:

- 1 red onion, chopped
- 1 pound beef stew meat, ground
- ½ teaspoon chili powder
- 1 egg, whisked
- ½ teaspoon olive oil
- ½ teaspoon sweet paprika
- 2 tablespoons white flour
- ½ teaspoon oregano, chopped

- ½ tablespoon basil, chopped

- A pinch of salt and black pepper

- ½ teaspoon marjoram, dried

Directions:

1. In a bowl, mix the beef with the onion, chili powder and the other ingredients except the oil, stir well and shape your meatloaf.

2. Grease a loaf pan that fits your slow cooker with the oil, add meatloaf mix into the pan, put it in your slow cooker, put the lid on and cook on Low for 4 hours.

3. Slice and serve for breakfast.

Nutrition: calories 200, fat 6, fiber 12, carbs 17, protein 10

Butternut Squash Quinoa

Preparation time: 10 minutes

Cooking time: 6 hours

Servings: 6

Ingredients:

- 1 yellow onion, chopped

- 1 tablespoon olive oil

- 3 garlic cloves, minced

- 2 teaspoons oregano, dried

- 1 and ½ pound chicken breasts, skinless, boneless and chopped

- 2 teaspoons parsley, dried

- 2 teaspoons curry powder

- ½ teaspoon chili flakes

- Salt and black pepper to the taste

- 1 butternut squash, peeled and cubed

- 2/3 cup quinoa

- 12 ounces canned tomatoes, chopped

- 4 cups veggie stock

Directions:

1. In your Slow cooker, mix onion with oil, garlic, oregano, chicken, parsley, curry powder, chili, squash, quinoa, salt, pepper, tomatoes and stock, stir, cover and cook on Low for 6 hours.

2. Divide into bowls and serve for breakfast.

Nutrition: calories 231, fat 4, fiber 6, carbs 20, protein 5

Leek Casserole

Preparation time: 10 minutes

Cooking time: 4 hours

Servings: 2

Ingredients:

- 1 cup leek, chopped
- Cooking spray
- ½ cup mozzarella, shredded
- 1 garlic clove, minced
- 4 eggs, whisked
- 1 cup beef sausage, chopped
- 1 tablespoon cilantro, chopped

Directions:

1. Grease the slow cooker with the cooking spray and mix the leek with the mozzarella and the other ingredients inside.

2. Toss, spread into the pot, put the lid on and cook on Low for 4 hours.

3. Divide between plates and serve for breakfast.

Nutrition: calories 232, fat 4, fiber 8, carbs 17, protein 4

Chia Seeds Mix

Preparation time: 10 minutes

Cooking time: 8 hours

Servings: 4

Ingredients:

- 1 cup steel cut oats
- 1 cup water
- 3 cups almond milk
- 2 tablespoons chia seeds
- ¼ cup pomegranate seeds
- ¼ cup dried blueberries
- ¼ cup almonds, sliced

Directions:

1. In your Slow cooker, mix oats with water, almond milk, chia seeds, pomegranate ones, blueberries and almonds, stir, cover and cook on Low for 8 hours.

2. Stir again, divide into bowls and serve for breakfast.

Nutrition: calories 200, fat 3, fiber 7, carbs 16, protein 3

Eggs and Sweet Potato Mix

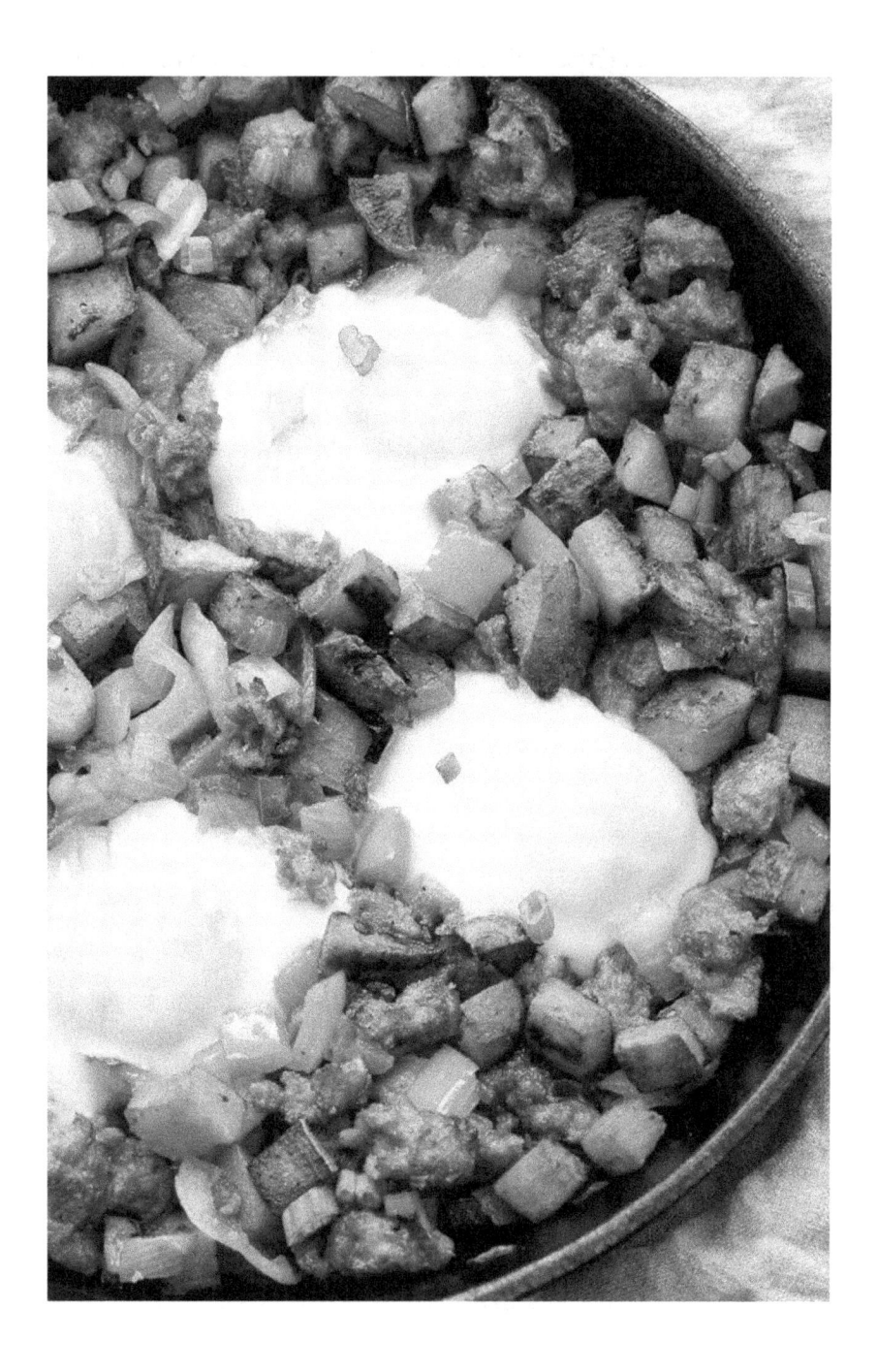

Preparation time: 10 minutes

Cooking time: 6 hours

Servings: 2

Ingredients:

- ½ red onion, chopped
- ½ green bell pepper, chopped
- 2 sweet potatoes, peeled and grated
- ½ red bell pepper, chopped
- 1 garlic clove, minced
- ½ teaspoon olive oil
- 4 eggs, whisked
- 1 tablespoon chives, chopped
- A pinch of red pepper, crushed
- A pinch of salt and black pepper

Directions:

1. In a bowl, mix the eggs with the onion, bell peppers and the other ingredients except the oil and whisk well.

2. Grease your slow cooker with the oil, add the eggs and potato mix, spread, put the lid on and cook on Low for 6 hours.

3. Divide everything between plates and serve.

Nutrition: calories 261, fat 6, fiber 6, carbs 16, protein 4

Chia Seeds and Chicken Breakfast

Preparation time: 10 minutes

Cooking time: 3 hours

Servings: 4

Ingredients:

- 1 pound chicken breasts, skinless, boneless and cubed
- ½ teaspoon basil, dried
- ¾ cup flaxseed, ground
- ¼ cup chia seeds
- ¼ cup parmesan, grated
- ½ teaspoon oregano, chopped
- Salt and black pepper to the taste
- 2 eggs

- 2 garlic cloves, minced

Directions:

1. In a bowl, mix flaxseed with chia seeds, parmesan, salt, pepper, oregano, garlic and basil and stir.

2. Put the eggs in a second bowl and whisk them well.

3. Dip chicken in eggs mix, then in chia seeds mix, put them in your Slow cooker after you've greased it with cooking spray, cover and cook on High for 3 hours.

4. Serve them right away for a Sunday breakfast.

Nutrition: calories 212, fat 3, fiber 4, carbs 17, protein 4

Pork and Eggplant Casserole

Preparation time: 10 minutes

Cooking time: 6 hours

Servings: 2

Ingredients:

- 1 red onion, chopped
- 1 eggplant, cubed
- ½ pound pork stew meat, ground
- 3 eggs, whisked
- ½ teaspoon chili powder
- ½ teaspoon garam masala
- 1 tablespoon sweet paprika
- 1 teaspoon olive oil

Directions:

1. In a bowl, mix the eggs with the meat, onion, eggplant and the other ingredients except the oil and stir well.

2. Grease your slow cooker with oil, add the pork and eggplant mix, spread into the pot, put the lid on and cook on Low for 6 hours.

3. Divide the mix between plates and serve for breakfast.

Nutrition: calories 261, fat 7, fiber 6, carbs 16, protein 7

Chocolate Quinoa

Preparation time: 10 minutes

Cooking time: 6 hours

Servings: 4

Ingredients:

- 1 cup quinoa
- 1 cup coconut milk
- 1 cup milk
- 2 tablespoons cocoa powder
- 3 tablespoons maple syrup
- 4 dark chocolate squares, chopped

Directions:

1. In your Slow cooker, mix quinoa with coconut milk, milk, cocoa powder, maple syrup and chocolate, stir, cover and cook on Low for 6 hours.

2. Stir quinoa mix again, divide into bowls and serve.

Nutrition: calories 215, fat 5, fiber 8, carbs 17, protein 4

Apple Spread

Preparation time: 10 minutes

Cooking time: 4 hours

Servings: 2

Ingredients:

- 2 apples, cored, peeled and pureed
- ½ cup coconut cream
- 2 tablespoons apple cider
- 2 tablespoons sugar
- ¼ teaspoon cinnamon powder
- ½ teaspoon lemon juice
- ¼ teaspoon ginger, grated

Directions:

1. In your slow cooker, mix the apple puree with the cream, sugar and the other ingredients, whisk, put the lid on and cook on High for 4 hours.

2. Blend using an immersion blender, cool down and serve for breakfast.

Nutrition: calories 172, fat 3, fiber 3, carbs 8, protein 3

Chai Breakfast Quinoa

Preparation time: 10 minutes

Cooking time: 6 hours

Servings: 2

Ingredients:

- 1 cup quinoa
- 1 egg white
- 2 cups milk
- ¼ teaspoon vanilla extract
- 1 and ½ tablespoons brown sugar
- ¼ teaspoon cardamom, ground
- ¼ teaspoon ginger, grated
- ¼ teaspoon cinnamon powder

- ¼ teaspoon vanilla extract

- ¼ teaspoon nutmeg, ground

- 1 tablespoons coconut flakes

Directions:

1. In your Slow cooker, mix quinoa with egg white, milk, vanilla, sugar, cardamom, ginger, cinnamon, vanilla and nutmeg, stir a bit, cover and cook on Low for 6 hours.

2. Stir, divide into bowls and serve for breakfast with coconut flakes on top.

Nutrition: calories 211, fat 4, fiber 6, carbs 10, protein 4

Cherries and Cocoa Oats

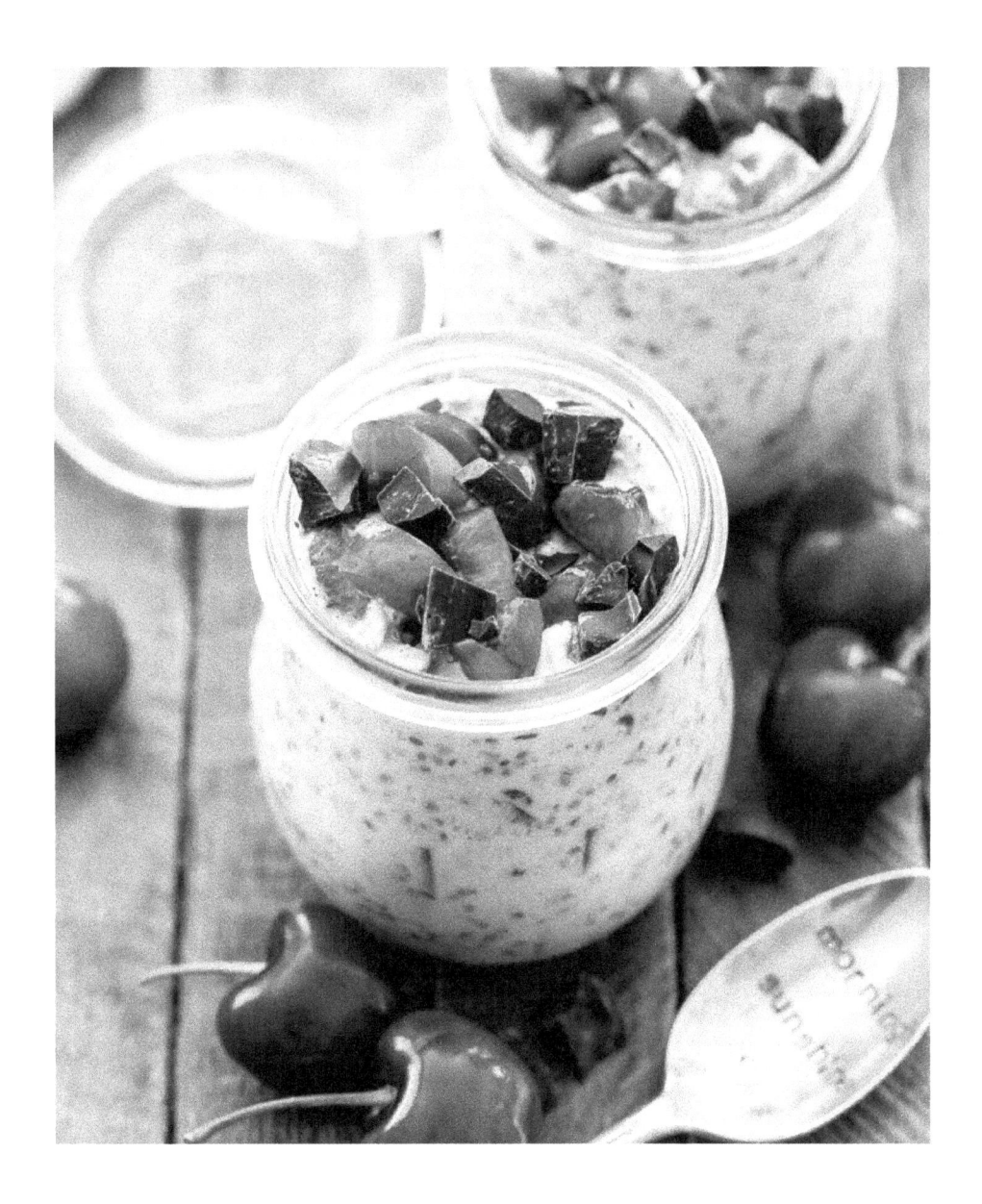

Preparation time: 10 minutes

Cooking time: 7 hours

Servings: 2

Ingredients:

- 1 cup almond milk
- ½ cup steel cut oats
- 1 tablespoon cocoa powder
- ½ cup cherries, pitted
- 2 tablespoons sugar
- ¼ teaspoon vanilla extract

Directions:

1. In your slow cooker, mix the almond milk with the cherries and the other ingredients, toss, put the lid on and cook on Low for 7 hours.
2. Divide into 2 bowls and serve for breakfast.

Nutrition: calories 150, fat 1, fiber 2, carbs 6, protein 5

Quinoa Breakfast Bake

Preparation time: 10 minutes

Cooking time: 7 hours

Servings: 4

Ingredients:

- 1 cup quinoa
- 4 tablespoons olive oil
- 2 cups water
- ½ cup dates, chopped
- 3 bananas, chopped
- ¼ cup coconut, shredded
- 2 teaspoons cinnamon powder
- 2 tablespoons brown sugar

- 1 cup walnuts, toasted and chopped

Directions:

1. Put the oil in your Slow cooker, add quinoa, water, dates, bananas, coconut, cinnamon, brown sugar and walnuts, stir, cover and cook on Low for 7 hours.

2. Divide into bowls and serve for breakfast.

Nutrition: calories 241, fat 4, fiber 8, carbs 16, protein 6

Beans Salad

Preparation time: 10 minutes

Cooking time: 6 hours

Servings: 2

Ingredients:

- 1 cup canned black beans, drained
- 1 cup canned red kidney beans, drained
- 1 cup baby spinach
- 2 spring onions, chopped
- ½ red bell pepper, chopped
- ¼ teaspoon turmeric powder
- ½ teaspoon garam masala
- ¼ cup veggie stock

- A pinch of cumin, ground

- A pinch of chili powder

- A pinch of salt and black pepper

- ½ cup salsa

Directions:

1. In your slow cooker, mix the beans with the spinach, onions and the other ingredients, toss, put the lid on and cook on High for 6 hours.

2. Divide the mix into bowls and serve for breakfast.

Nutrition: calories 130, fat 4, fiber 2, carbs 5, protein 4

Mocha Latte Quinoa Mix

Preparation time: 10 minutes

Cooking time: 6 hours

Servings: 4

Ingredients:

- 1 cup hot coffee
- 1 cup quinoa
- 1 cup coconut water
- ¼ cup chocolate chips
- ½ cup coconut cream

Directions:

1. In your Slow cooker, mix quinoa with coffee, coconut water and chocolate chips, cover and cook on Low for 6 hours.

2. Stir, divide into bowls, spread coconut cream all over and serve for breakfast.

Nutrition: calories 251, fat 4, fiber 7, carbs 15, protein 4

Peppers Rice Mix

Preparation time: 10 minutes

Cooking time: 3 hours

Servings: 2

Ingredients:

- ½ cup brown rice
- 1 cup chicken stock
- 2 spring onions, chopped
- ½ orange bell pepper, chopped
- ½ red bell pepper, chopped
- ½ green bell pepper, chopped
- 2 ounces canned green chilies, chopped
- ½ cup canned black beans, drained

- ½ cup mild salsa

- ½ teaspoon sweet paprika

- ½ teaspoon lime zest, grated

- A pinch of salt and black pepper

Directions:

1. In your slow cooker, mix the rice with the stock, spring onions and the other ingredients, toss, put the lid on and cook on High for 3 hours.

2. Divide the mix into bowls and serve for breakfast.

Nutrition: calories 140, fat 2, fiber 2, carbs 5, protein 5

Breakfast Butterscotch Pudding

Preparation time: 10 minutes

Cooking time: 1 hour and 40 minutes

Servings: 6

Ingredients:

- 4 ounces butter, melted
- 2 ounces brown sugar
- 7 ounces flour
- ¼ pint milk
- 1 teaspoon vanilla extract
- Zest of ½ lemon, grated
- 2 tablespoons maple syrup
- Cooking spray

- 1 egg

Directions:

1. In a bowl, mix butter with sugar, milk, vanilla, lemon zest, maple syrup and eggs and whisk well.

2. Add flour and whisk really well again.

3. Grease your Slow cooker with cooking spray, add pudding mix, spread, cover and cook on High for 1 hour and 30 minutes.

4. Divide between plates and serve for breakfast.

Nutrition: calories 271, fat 5, fiber 5, carbs 17, protein 4

Cashew Butter

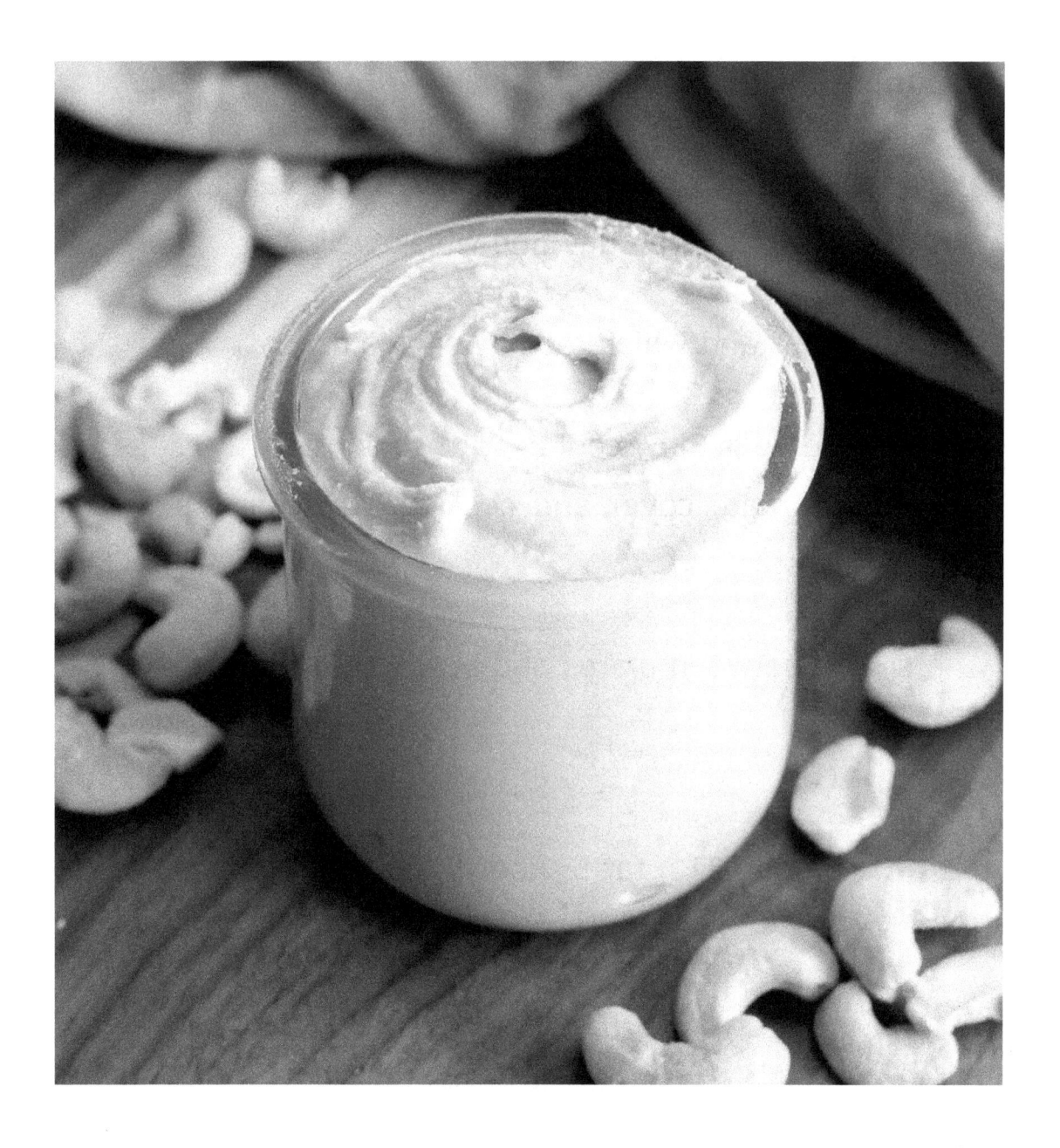

Preparation time: 10 minutes

Cooking time: 4 hours

Servings: 2

Ingredients:

- 1 cup cashews, soaked overnight, drained and blended
- ½ cup coconut cream
- ¼ teaspoon cinnamon powder
- 1 teaspoon lemon zest, grated
- 2 tablespoons sugar
- A pinch of ginger, ground

Directions:

1. In your slow cooker, mix the cashews with the cream and the other ingredients, whisk, put the lid on and cook on High for 4 hours.
2. Blend using an immersion blender, divide into jars, and serve for breakfast cold.

Nutrition: calories 143, fat 2, fiber 3, carbs 3, protein 4

French Breakfast Pudding

Preparation time: 10 minutes

Cooking time: 1 hour and 30 minutes

Servings: 4

Ingredients:

- 3 egg yolks

- 6 ounces double cream

- 1 teaspoon vanilla extract

- 2 tablespoons caster sugar

Directions:

1. In a bowl, mix the egg yolks with sugar and whisk well.

2. Add cream and vanilla extract, whisk well, pour into your 4 ramekins, place them in your Slow cooker, add some water to the slow cooker, cover and cook on High for 1 hour and 30 minutes.

3. Leave aside to cool down and serve.

Nutrition: calories 261, fat 5, fiber 6, carbs 15, protein 2

Pumpkin and Berries Bowls

Preparation time: 10 minutes

Cooking time: 4 hours

Servings: 2

Ingredients:

- ½ cup coconut cream
- 1 and ½ cups pumpkin, peeled and cubed
- 1 cup blackberries
- 2 tablespoons maple syrup
- ¼ teaspoon nutmeg, ground
- ½ teaspoon vanilla extract

Directions:

1. In your slow cooker, combine the pumpkin with the berries, cream and the other ingredients, toss, put the lid on and cook on Low for 4 hours.

2. Divide into bowls and serve for breakfast!

Nutrition: calories 120, fat 2, fiber 2, carbs 4, protein 2

Eggs and Sausage Casserole

Preparation time: 10 minutes

Cooking time: 8 hours

Servings: 4

Ingredients:

- 8 eggs, whisked
- 1 yellow onion, chopped
- 1 pound pork sausage, chopped
- 2 teaspoons basil, dried
- 1 tablespoon garlic powder
- Salt and black pepper to the taste
- 1 yellow bell pepper, chopped
- 1 teaspoon olive oil

Directions:

1. Grease your Slow cooker with the olive oil, add eggs, onion, pork sausage, basil, garlic powder, salt, pepper and yellow bell pepper, toss, cover and cook on Low for 8 hours.

2. Slice, divide between plates and serve for breakfast.

Nutrition: calories 301, fat 4, fiber 4, carbs 14, protein 7

Quinoa and Chia Pudding

Preparation time: 10 minutes

Cooking time: 6 hours

Servings: 2

Ingredients:

- 1 cup coconut cream
- 2 tablespoons chia seeds
- ½ cup almond milk
- 1 tablespoon sugar
- ½ cup quinoa, rinsed
- ½ teaspoon vanilla extract

Directions:

1. In your slow cooker, mix the cream with the chia seeds and the other ingredients, toss, put the lid on and cook on Low for 6 hours.

2. Divide into 2 bowls and serve for breakfast.

Nutrition: calories 120, fat 2, fiber 1, carbs 6, protein 4

Cauliflower Rice Pudding

Preparation time: 10 minutes

Cooking time: 2 hours

Servings: 2

Ingredients:

- ¼ cup maple syrup
- 3 cups almond milk
- 1 cup cauliflower rice
- 2 tablespoons vanilla extract

Directions:

1. Put cauliflower rice in your Slow cooker, add maple syrup, almond milk and vanilla extract, stir, cover and cook on High for 2 hours.

2. Stir your pudding again, divide into bowls and serve for breakfast.

Nutrition: calories 240, fat 2, fiber 2, carbs 15, protein 5

Beans Breakfast Bowls

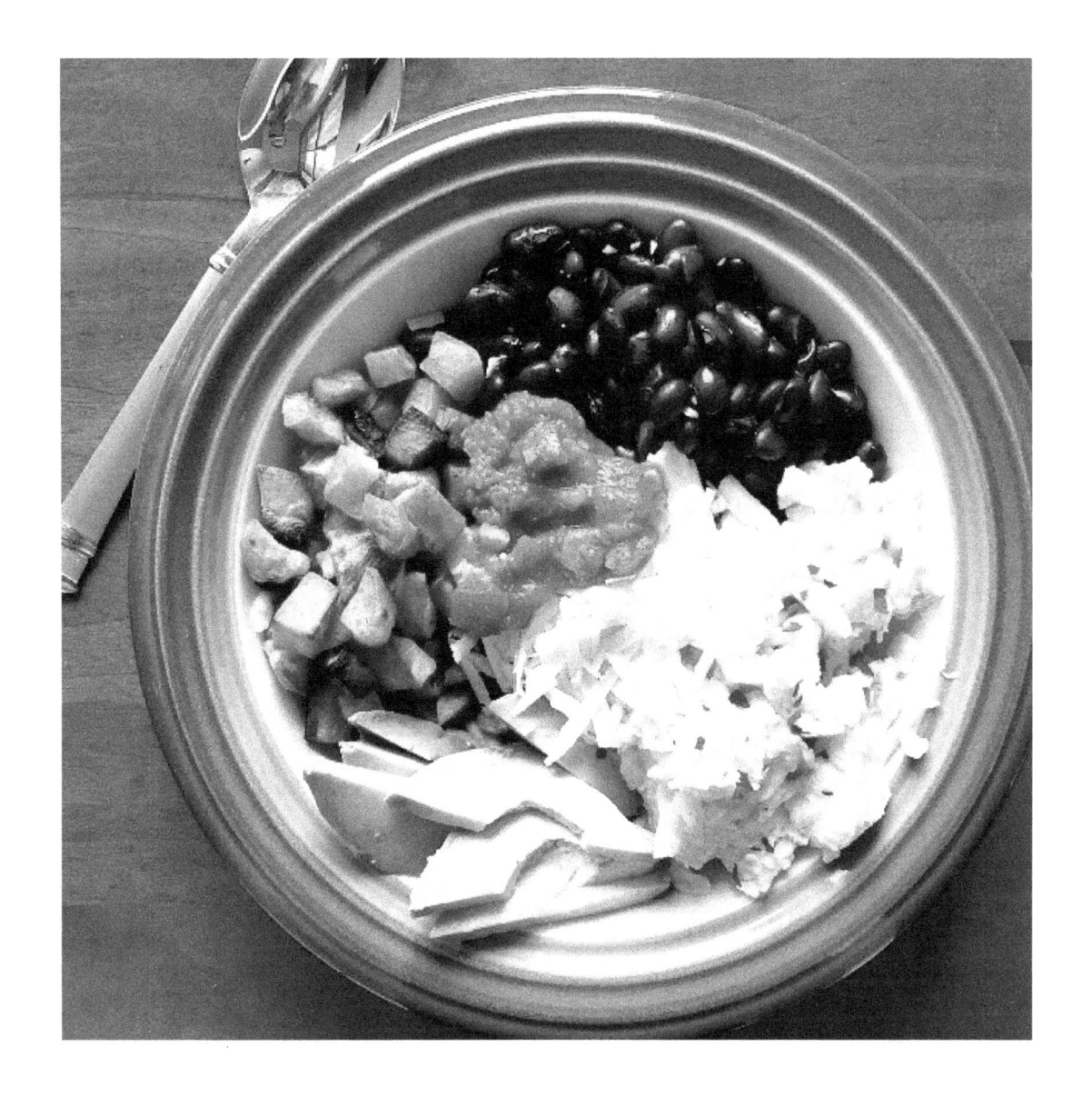

Preparation time: 10 minutes

Cooking time: 3 hours and 10 minutes

Servings: 2

Ingredients:

- 2 spring onions, chopped
- ½ green bell pepper, chopped
- ½ red bell pepper, chopped
- ½ yellow onion, chopped
- 5 ounces canned black beans, drained
- 5 ounces canned red kidney beans, drained
- 5 ounces canned pinto beans, drained
- ½ cup corn
- ½ teaspoon turmeric powder
- 1 teaspoons chili powder
- ½ teaspoon hot sauce
- A pinch of salt and black pepper
- 1 tablespoon olive oil

Directions:

1. Heat up a pan with the oil over medium-high heat, add the spring onions, bell peppers and the onion, sauté for 10 minutes and transfer to the slow cooker.

2. Add the beans and the other ingredients, toss, put the lid on and cook on High for 3 hours.

3. Divide the mix into bowls and serve for breakfast.

Nutrition: calories 240, fat 4, fiber 2, carbs 6, protein 9

Conclusion

Did you indulge in attempting these new and tasty dishes? regrettably we have come to the end of this sluggish stove cookbook, I really wish it has actually been to your liking. to increase your health and health we would certainly enjoy to recommend you to integrate exercise as well as likewise a dynamic method of living together with adhere to these outstanding dishes, so as to highlight the improvements. we will certainly be back soon with other significantly intriguing vegan dishes, a big hug, see you quickly.

CPSIA information can be obtained
at www.ICGtesting.com
Printed in the USA
LVHW102020020621
689027LV00009BA/926